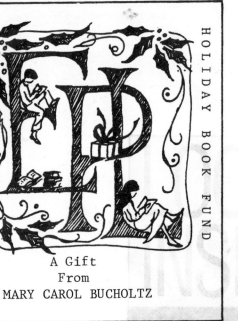
LOOKING INSIDE

SPORTS Aerodynamics

Ron Schultz

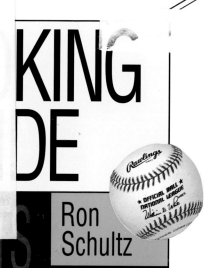

ILLUSTRATED BY
Peter Aschwanden
and
Nick Gadbois

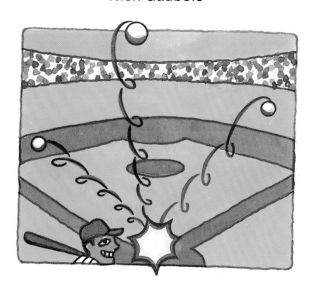

John Muir Publications
Santa Fe, New Mexico

John Muir Publications, P.O. Box 613, Santa Fe, NM 87504

First edition. First printing September 1992

Library of Congress Cataloging-in-Publication Data
Schultz, Ron (Ronald), 1951-
    Looking inside sports aerodynamics / Ron Schultz
    — 1st ed.
      p. cm.
    Includes index
    Summary: Explains the principles of aerodynamic forces and
how they function in such sports as tennis, football, baseball,
track and field, and golf.
    ISBN 1-56261-065-1 (paper)
    1. Dynamics—Juvenile literature. 2. Aerodynamics—Juvenile
literature. 3. Force and energy—Juvenile literature.
[1. Dynamics. 2. Aerodynamics. 3. Force and energy. 4. Sports.]
I. Title
QC133.5.S38   1992
796'.01'53362—dc20

                                    92-4957
                                    CIP
                                    AC

Design: Ken Wilson
Photography: Sports Chrome West, Inc.; Spalding Sports Worldwide;
    John Reed, Wilson Sporting Goods; FRISBEE® disc (FRISBEE® is a
    brand name and a registered trademark of Kransco); Rawlings®.
Illustrations: Nick Gadbois, Peter Aschwanden
Typeface: New Century Schoolbook, Princetown
Typography: Ken Wilson
Printer: Inland Press

Distributed to the book trade by
W. W. Norton & Company, Inc.
New York, New York

Distributed to the education market by
The Wright Group
19201 120th Avenue NE
Bothell, WA 98011

I would like to express my grateful appreciation to the following people for their open phone lines and their excellent information: Mike Sullivan and Pam Stone from Spalding Sports, Frank Garrett from Wilson Sports, Frank Kappler of Wham-O, Bob Myers from the University of Arizona, and Sharon Smith at the LANL Library. In addition, my special appreciation goes to the people at John Muir Publications for their vision and patience and to Laura Sanderford for her daily support, insights and contributions.

This book is dedicated to the memory of Steven T. Howell A great sports fan

CONTENTS

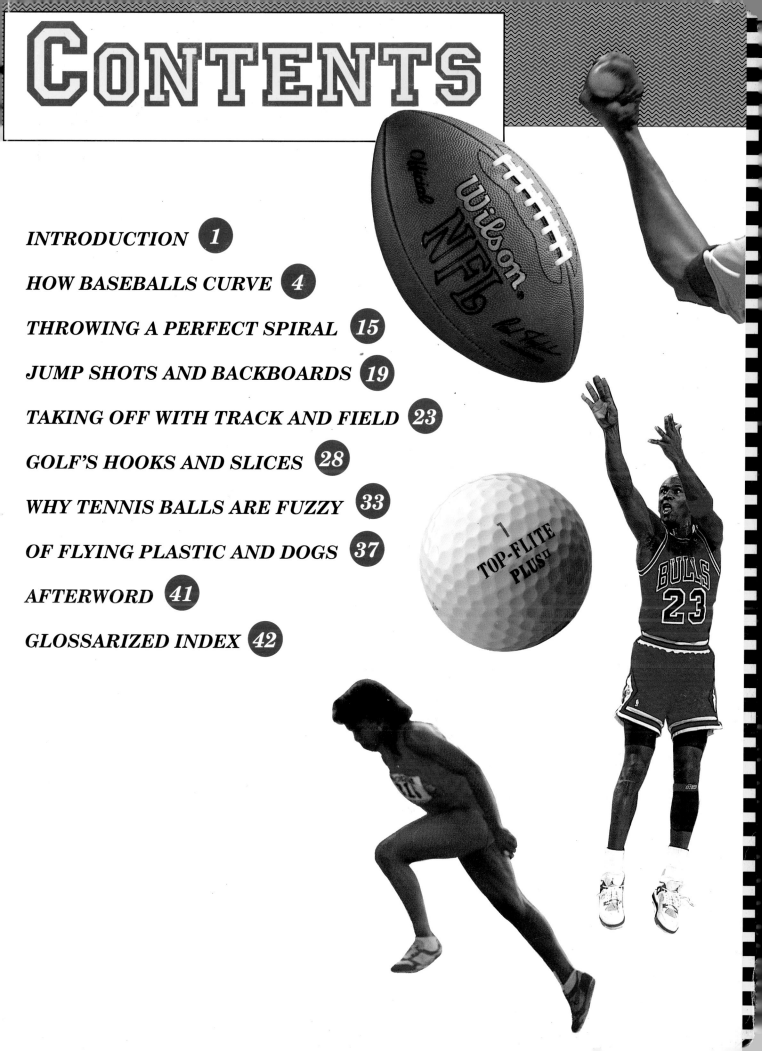

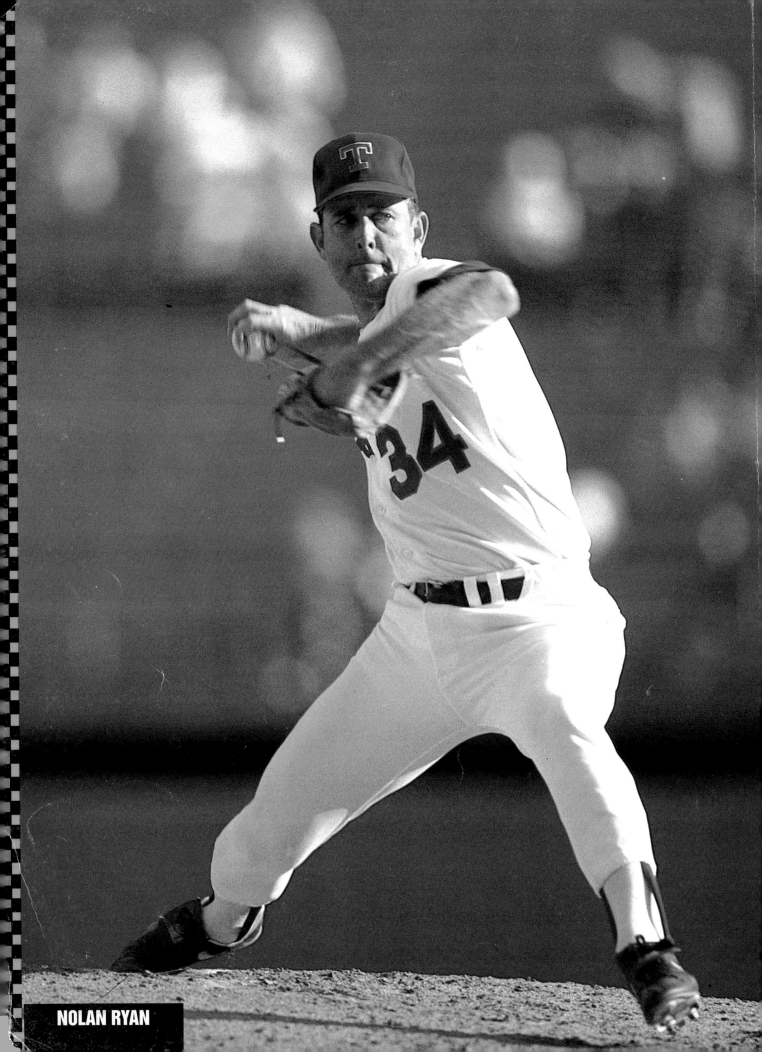

NOLAN RYAN

INTRODUCTION

Sports require an amazing amount of swooping, sailing, and skidding through the air. With or without the benefit of an air traffic controller, all air travel is governed by the forces of aerodynamics. Basically, "aero" means air, and "dynamics" means how things move. So aerodynamics is how things move in the air. How airplanes, birds, and rockets fly. How winds blow. How knuckleballs flutter. How basketballs swish through the hoop. How a golf ball sails toward the hole.

We are about to take off on an aerial display of how baseballs, footballs, basketballs, tennis balls, golf balls, people, Frisbees, and even Frisbee-catching dogs dip, spin, flutter, float, and slice through the air with the greatest of ease. So let's fasten our seat belts, sports fans. We have just been given our final clearance for takeoff.

ALL ABOUT AIR

The air we live in and breathe is actually a fluid. It doesn't look like water, it's true. But, like water, it's made up of billions of gas molecules that are constantly on the move. These molecules bombard everything they encounter. And when they hit a surface, they bounce back.

One of the reasons we move through air so easily is that it can be squished, squeezed, and compressed into almost any shape. Like the elastic that holds up a basketball player's shorts, air expands and contracts in any and all directions. Air can do this because of all the open space between the floating molecules.

All the hitting and bouncing back that air molecules do builds up a force called pressure, so we have what is known as *air* pressure. Squeezing makes more air pressure. So does weight. Imagine that these floating molecules are stacked one on top of another in a great layer that surrounds the earth. At sea level, all the air molecules on top press down on the air molecules below them. Because of this pressing down, air pressure is greater at sea level. At higher altitudes, there isn't so much pressing down (and thus not so much weight), so air pressure is less.

KIRBY PUCKETT

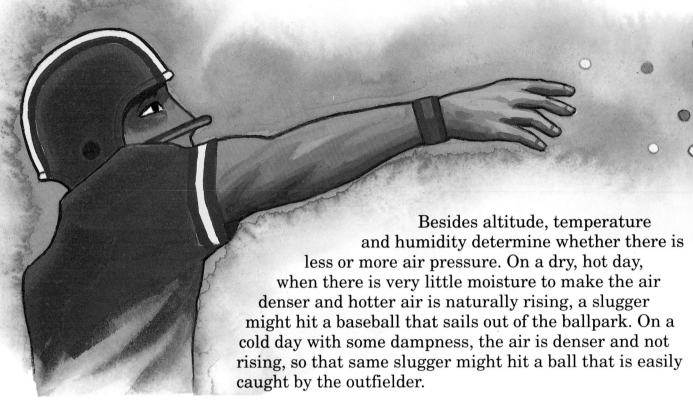

Besides altitude, temperature and humidity determine whether there is less or more air pressure. On a dry, hot day, when there is very little moisture to make the air denser and hotter air is naturally rising, a slugger might hit a baseball that sails out of the ballpark. On a cold day with some dampness, the air is denser and not rising, so that same slugger might hit a ball that is easily caught by the outfielder.

NICK GADBOIS

FOR THE BIRDS

Centuries ago, people got the idea by watching birds in flight, that air *pushed* objects along. It wasn't until the fifteenth century that Leonardo da Vinci, who never once threw a football, discovered that air actually offered resistance to things moving through it. Da Vinci figured that air resisted because all the air molecules were compressed as they met the object in flight. When the object squished the air in front of it, it made it denser—and also heavier. This heavy air made it more difficult, rather than easier, for flying objects to move through it.

In the seventeenth century, Sir Isaac Newton, of falling apple fame, gave us the concept of gravity—a force of attraction between bodies. For our purposes here, this is simply: what goes up, must come down. To stay in the air, objects must overcome gravity. But more about that later.

BUMPS IN THE AIRSTREAM

Modern aerodynamics really took off in the twentieth century. The Wright brothers, the dynamic duo who were the first men to fly, were major contributors. What they and others discovered were the effects of *turbulence, drag,* and *lift.*

Air flows in two ways. One way is in smooth layers. This is when all the "streamlines" of air are flowing together. The second way is when the streamlines of air are broken or choppy. If you've ever experienced a bumpy airplane ride, you know all about this. Those bumps are sections of the airstream that are going in different directions, and they are called turbulence.

Drag isn't just something that is boring to do or a person you

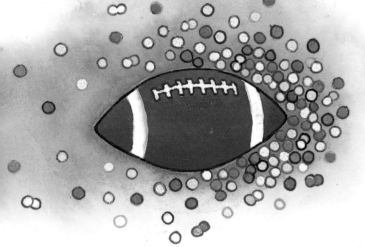

A football compresses the air it meets

don't want to be with. It's also the resistance an object meets from the air it travels through. If you were to stick your hand out the window of a car while driving down the street, it would be forced back by the air flowing around it. That's drag. All objects, even baseballs, basketballs, golf balls, and tennis balls, have to struggle against the effects of drag.

You might think that since a ball is round, the drag would not be as strong, that the air would slip around it. But that's not so. Remember, air is a fluid, and it actually sticks to the ball. This stickiness creates another kind of drag, friction. A ball traveling through the air faces double drag—from air pressure and from friction.

As we will see, the drag on a ball affects how it moves through the air. And drag, itself, is affected by things like stitches, seams, bumps, holes, and fuzz.

The final ingredient in the sports aerodynamics equation is lift. A batted baseball can't sail over the outfield fence unless it has been able to rise through the air. A pitcher throws the ball toward the batter. The batter swings the bat and smashes the ball in the opposite direction. The force of the pitch combined with the force of the bat overcome the weight of the ball (remember gravity), so the ball sails off the bat, rising like an airplane taking off. As we will see, the shape of the ball, together with its spinning, allows air to move faster over it than underneath it. This means there is less air pressure on top and greater air pressure underneath. That greater air pressure pushes the ball up.

We'll explain more about how air pressure, air resistance, lift, and speed work together to produce home runs, touchdowns, and holes-in-one.

You might think that air moving over the top of an object faster than it is moving underneath it should push that object down, rather than lift it up. But it doesn't. There is a simple experiment that shows this aerodynamic principle in action. Take a long narrow piece of paper and hold it so it bends over your finger. Then blow over the top of it. The paper will rise. What is happening is that the air flowing over the top of the paper decreases the air pressure that is pushing down on the paper and increases the air pressure pushing up from underneath. If the pressure pushing up from underneath is greater than the pressure pushing down on it from on top, the object will rise.

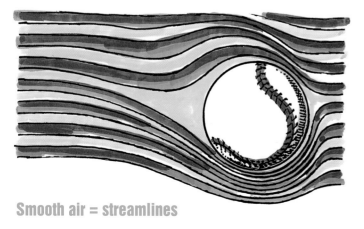

Smooth air = streamlines

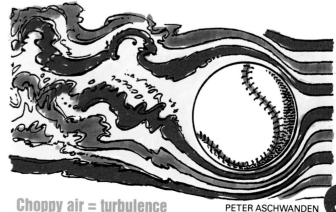

Choppy air = turbulence

PETER ASCHWANDEN

HOW BASEBALLS CURVE

"The count to Will Clark is 3 and 2. The Giants have runners on the corners, and they're trailing the Mets 4 to 3 with two out in the bottom of the ninth. Doc Gooden is on the mound for the Mets. He stares down for the sign. Clark waves the bat behind his left ear, waiting for the pitch. Gooden rocks into his windup, and here's the 3-2 pitch. Clark swings and misses, as Gooden breaks off a dandy curveball that has Clark swinging at ball four in the dirt. I tell you, folks, that curveball looked like it fell off the edge of a table. . ."

Ever since pitchers began throwing baseballs overhand in 1884, curveballs have been fooling batters, left and right. Pitchers scratched, scuffed, and loaded up the ball with all kinds of sticky stuff like spit and Vaseline to make it dance and dive on its way toward the batter. This stuff made the air push against the ball in places it normally wouldn't, creating greater air resistance as it made its way to home plate. This caused the ball to travel erratically, so the hitter wasn't quite sure just where it would cross the plate. It was during this time that baseball changed from a hitter's game to a pitcher's game.

INSIDE BASEBALL

After the 1919 season, applying foreign substances to the ball or scratching or scuffing it in any way was made illegal. To regain their advantage, pitchers began applying *spin* to the ball to make it change direction.

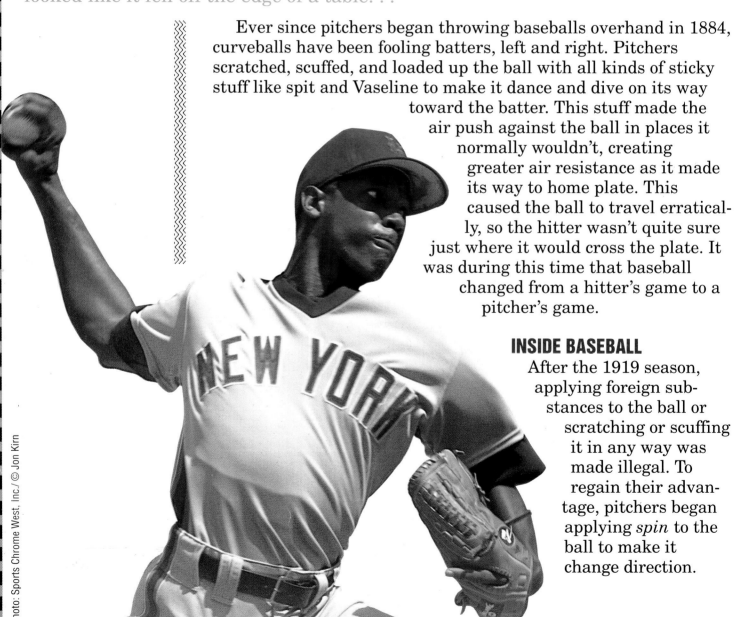

DWIGHT GOODEN

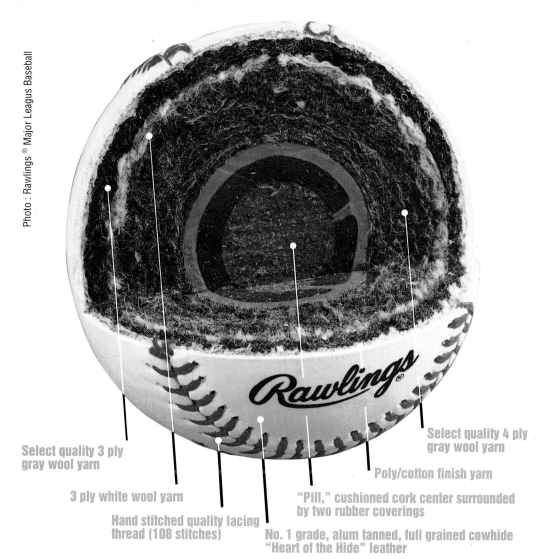

Select quality 3 ply
gray wool yarn

3 ply white wool yarn

Hand stitched quality lacing
thread (108 stitches)

"Pill," cushioned cork center surrounded
by two rubber coverings

No. 1 grade, alum tanned, full grained cowhide
"Heart of the Hide" leather

Poly/cotton finish yarn

Select quality 4 ply
gray wool yarn

Before we describe how a baseball curves and dips through the air legally, let's first describe the ball itself. It's round, and at its center is a small sphere of cork or rubber surrounded by yarn. The yarn is covered by 2 strips of white horsehide or cowhide. The baseball weighs between 5 and 5½ ounces, and it's between 9 and 9¼ inches around. And, last but certainly not least, the covering of the ball has exactly 108 raised cotton stitches.

The flight of a baseball is primarily affected by those 5 ounces of yarn and cowhide—the ball's weight—combined with the speed at which the ball is thrown or batted. The main aerodynamic factors working against the flight of the ball are air resistance and its good buddy, drag.

WILL CLARK

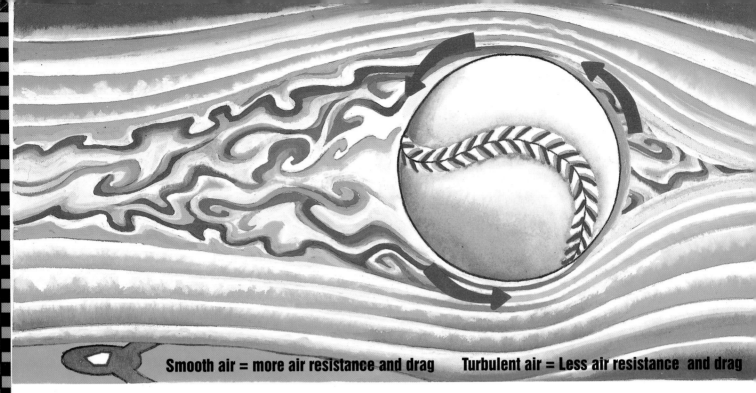

THE WINDUP! THE PITCH!

During a game, the baseball travels at a speed of somewhere between 50 and 120 miles per hour (mph). At a slower speed, the air around the ball is pretty smooth. The ball pushes against the smooth air, easily compressing it and creating a lot of air resistance. When the ball travels faster, it causes the air to be more turbulent, and there's *less* air resistance. The 108 spinning stitches of the baseball help the ball move the air. They break up the air. So air molecules don't form as great a barrier to the ball. If the ball were perfectly smooth, it couldn't be thrown or hit as far, because it would be unable to break up the air resistance it met.

The direction and speed of the spinning stitches also affect the drag on the ball. The faster the spin, the less the drag. The slower the spin, the greater the drag. The reason for this is the stitches catch the air around the ball as it moves through the air. The drag effects on a pitched ball are slight, since it takes less than half a second for a baseball going 50 to 100 mph to get from the pitcher to the catcher. As we will see, there is more drag on a batted ball than on a pitched ball.

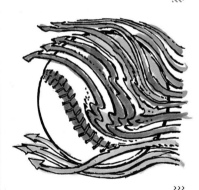

The effect of a baseball's seams on its flight

THE CURVEBALL

A pitcher usually throws a curveball by holding his index and middle fingers close together along the seam of the ball. He releases the ball just after it clears his ear. As the pitcher lets go of the ball, he snaps his fingers over the top of it so that it rolls over his middle finger. This snapping motion creates topspin. (It also creates a good deal of strain on the pitcher's elbow. For this reason, it is not recommended that little leaguers throw any kind of curveball. Leave the curveballs, screwballs, and sliders for the older boys.)

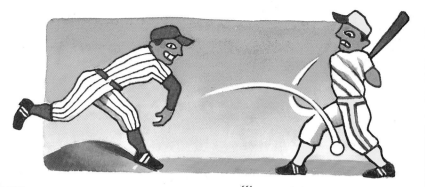

The stitches on a curveball spin at about 1,800 revolutions per minute (rpm). As they spin, the stitches catch the air and pull a thin layer of it around the ball. The spin pushes more air around the bottom than the top, which causes the bottom of the ball to move faster than the top, which creates less air pressure on the bottom. Together with the force of gravity, the greater air pressure on the top of the ball pushes the ball down and causes its curving motion. At 1,800 rpm, a curveball with topspin can curve as much as 17½ inches!

Down and Sideways

A curveball doesn't only curve down. If it is thrown sidearm, it will curve across the plate. In fact, if there were no gravity to pull the ball down, a pitcher might actually throw a sidearm curveball that would encircle an entire baseball stadium.

Contrary to what many batters say, the curveball follows a constant curve on its way from the pitcher to the catcher. It doesn't suddenly plunge. The arc of the ball does curve more toward the end of the pitch than when it leaves the pitcher's hand, but this is because of the distance involved and the laws of gravity.

That is not how the batter sees it. When the ball leaves the pitcher's hand, it looks flat and then seems to break at the last second and suddenly drop. This is why the downward spinning curveball is the most difficult to hit. It doesn't give the batter enough time to properly judge the level of his swing. The batter is likely to hit the top of the ball, rather than the middle. And when this happens, it's a ground ball.

So why does a batter think a curveball drops suddenly? Imagine you were watching a Ferris wheel from the side as it circled around. The chairs of the wheel seem to circle at an even rate. But if you were to stand right next to the wheel, the chairs would seem to speed up as they got closer to you. This same optical illusion is what happens to a batter facing a topspin curveball.

FIGURING EARNED RUN AVERAGES

One of the results of being able to throw a devastating curveball or a demonic split-finger fastball is that batters have a terrible time hitting them. This development tends to decrease a pitcher's earned run average (ERA). An ERA is the number of earned runs a pitcher allows, on average, during each 9 innings he pitches. To calculate a pitcher's ERA, take the number of innings pitched and divide that by 9. Then take the number of earned runs allowed (no error-produced runs please) and divide that by the number you arrived at in the first calculation, and you get the ERA. For example, Scott Erickson pitched 113 innings and allowed 36 earned runs. Dividing 113 by 9, we get 12.56. Dividing 36 by 12.56 gives us Erickson's ERA of 2.87 earned runs allowed per 9 innings.

Can you figure out Ramon Martinez's ERA? He pitched 234 innings and allowed 76 earned runs.

Answer: 2.92

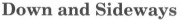

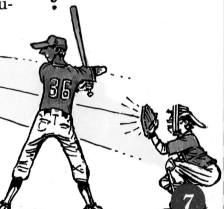

The drop of a curveball

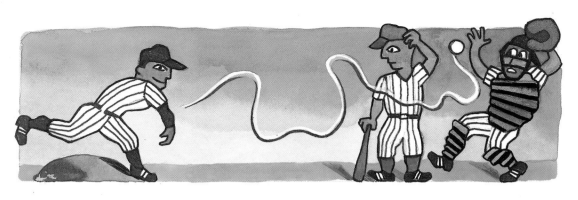

THE KNUCKLEBALL

It dances. It prances. It swoops. It dives. It moves right and left almost at the same time. It defies logic, catchers, pitchers, and hitters. It's the knuckleball. It makes hitters feel foolish and catchers wonder if maybe they should look for different work. Bob Uecker, a former major league catcher and now a TV personality, once said that the best way to catch a knuckleball was to "just wait until the ball stops rolling and pick it up."

There have not been a lot of knuckleballers in baseball, because it takes a *lot* of skill to throw consistently. Hoyt Willhelm was one of the greats. So were the Neikro brothers, Phil and Jim. When he was 43 years old, Phil won 17 games throwing the knuckler. Today, Charlie Hough, currently with the Texas Rangers, is the top knuckler. But it has taken years to perfect this pitch.

Oddly enough (but then nothing should be odd when talking about the knuckleball), the pitch is not thrown with the knuckles but with the fingertips. The object is to throw the ball with as little spin as possible. A knuckleball might reach a top speed of just 50 mph and spin only 1/4 revolution on its way to home plate. (Remember, the curveball can fly at up to *80* mph and spin *18* times on its way to home plate.)

On the Way to the Plate

This lack of spin and slow speed means that a knuckleball is subject to certain forces of aerodynamics that other balls don't

PHIL NEIKRO

have to contend with. Its very slight spin means that the way it faces home plate affects what will happen to it in flight.

The knuckleball is the only pitch in which aerodynamic influences change as the ball travels to home plate. If the smooth part of the ball is headed toward the batter, it may appear to go straight, but then as the ball rotates slightly, the air may push on a seam and send it off to the right. It is even possible for the ball to head toward the right and then shift toward the left.

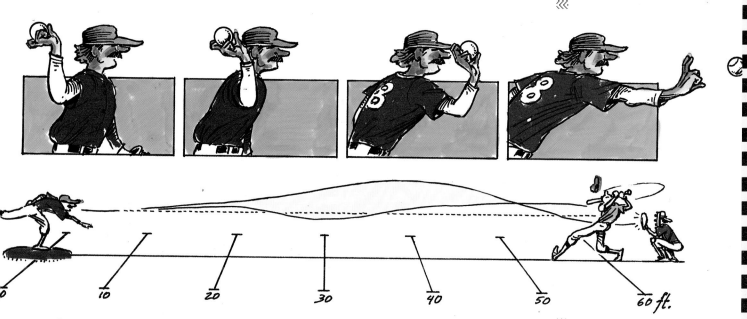

The ideal knuckleball has a *slight* spin. If there is too much spin, the aerodynamic effects are cancelled out. It is then just a slow bloop. The pitch quickly changes from a hitter's fright to a hitter's delight.

The crazy dance of the knuckleball

Drag also comes into play while the knuckleball is in flight. Since a knuckleball travels so slowly, it doesn't break up the air as much as a fast pitch. The smooth air, which is easily compressed, creates greater air resistance and a drag effect behind the ball, much like the wake that flows behind a ship at sea. This drag can be four times greater than the drag on a fastball. Pitchers have learned to take advantage of this. They release the ball at just the right speed so that halfway to home plate, the changeover to the smooth air takes place, and the ball slows down. Gravity takes over, and the ball suddenly drops.

It should be mentioned that the same dancing effects obtained by a knuckleball can also be achieved illegally with wet or greasy fingers. A spitball or Vaseline ball and a scuffed or cut ball will behave a lot like a knuckleball—but at a much faster speed. Because these pitches presented such an unfair advantage to the pitcher, they have been outlawed. Even so, some pitchers today are still able to slip them by an unsuspecting umpire and a baffled batter.

THE FIRE OF A FASTBALL

Throwing smoke, showing 'em the heater, burning it in there. Famous fastballers, Nolan Ryan, Roger Clemens, Sandy Koufax, Bob Feller, Goose Gossage, and Lefty Grove. All of them challenging hitters, rearing back and searing the air as they threw the ball as hard as they could: 99 mph, 100

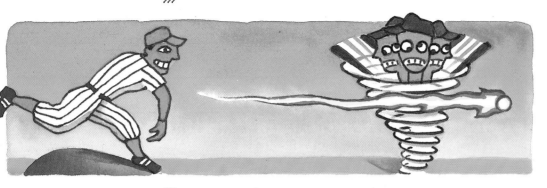

mph, 101 mph, making that 60'6" trip in under 0.4 second. For a batter to hit a pitch going that fast, his swing has to begin before the ball is even halfway to the plate. Because of drag, the ball is really going 8 mph faster when it leaves the pitcher's hand than when it arrives at home plate. Air resistance slows the ball 1 mph for every 7 feet it travels.

An overhand fastball is thrown with a good deal of backspin. Backspin is applied as the pitcher releases the ball. The downward motion of his fingers causes the ball to turn toward him. At 1,500 rpm, this backspin motion makes the ball rise or look like it "hops" slightly, the opposite optical illusion effect of a curveball. But like the curveball, the break in the pitch takes place about 15 feet before it reaches the batter.

The lift on a fastball is only about 4 to 5 inches. But that is just enough of a hop to fool a batter who has begun to swing his bat at the ball before it is even halfway to home plate.

Delivering the Heater

There are a number of different ways a pitcher can deliver a fastball. One is to place the fingers with the seams, so that *two* seams circle with each revolution of the ball. In the cross-seams technique, the pitcher's fingers are placed across the wide part of the seams, so *four* seams circle with each revolution. Because the with-the-seams fastball only shows two seams per revolution, its ride to home plate is smoother than the cross-seams fastball. The cross-seams fastball is about 5 mph faster than

ROGER CLEMENS

the with-the-seams fastball. This means if both pitches were thrown at the same time, as the cross-seams pitch crosses home plate, the with-the-seams pitch would be a foot and a half behind.

Because there is less drag on the cross-seams fastball, there is also less of an upward rise.

Some pitchers throw a sinking fastball. To do this, they move their fingers off the seams of the with-the-seams delivery and onto the

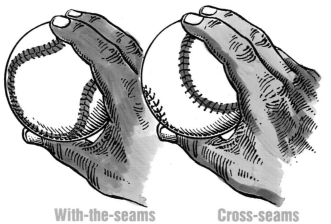

With-the-seams **Cross-seams**

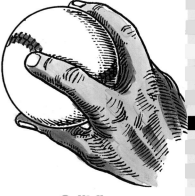

Split-finger

smooth leather. This allows the ball to spin less, which creates greater air resistance against it. By the time this fastball reaches home plate, it will be about 4 to 6 inches lower than the normal backspin rising fastball.

The split-finger fastball has made quite a hit lately. It was popularized by San Francisco Giants Manager Roger Craig. It uses the same delivery as a conventional fastball, but by spreading the fingers and holding the ball between the first and middle fingers at the first joint, a pitcher can throw the ball with much less spin. This pitch is also slightly slower, so it drops up to 10 inches more than the sinking fastball. Again, less spin, greater air resistance. If a conventional fastball and a split-fingered fastball were thrown at the same time, as the conventional fastball crossed home plate, the split-finger fastball would be 7 feet behind. This is a great advantage for a pitcher, since the batter's timing is based on the conventional fastball, and his swing will be partially completed by the time the ball arrives at home plate.

THE BATTER'S DILEMMA

George Brett, Wade Boggs, Ted Williams, Ty Cobb, Pete Rose, Tony Gwynn, Pedro Guerrero, and Kirby Puckett are all great hitters. And they have something in common: they make an out over two-thirds of the time! Baseball is probably the only game in which a player can fail 7 out of 10 times and still make the Hall of Fame as a great player. Making contact with a 9-inch circumference ball traveling at almost 100 mph from a distance of only 60'6" is not easy. But those aren't the only considerations: a batter must decide in a heartbeat the speed of the ball—fast, slow, or somewhere in between—and if it is going to curve away, sink, hop to his chest, jam him on the hands, slide outside, or flutter in three different directions before it gets to him. He must also decide if the pitch is inside or outside the strike zone. And all he has to defend himself with at the plate is a stick.

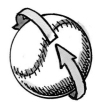

Fastball

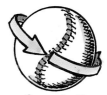

Curveball

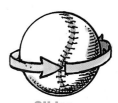

Slider

Screwball

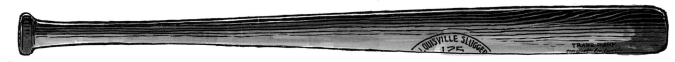

That stick has regulations of its own. According to the official rules of major league baseball, it must be smooth and rounded and not more than 2 inches in diameter at the thickest part. Also, it can't be more than 42 inches long. It can be one piece of solid wood or two or more pieces of wood bonded together. Aluminum bats, not allowed in the major leagues, follow all rules but the last.

The Swing

To describe what happens when the bat and ball come together, let's look at two different kinds of batters: first, Eric Davis, a right-handed towering home run hitter; second, Tony Gwynn, a left-handed, high-average, line-drive base hit artist. Both are excellent at doing what they do—Gwynn at getting a hit, Davis at hitting the ball over the fence.

Both batters hold the bat fairly upright. When the ball is about halfway between the mound and home plate, they both step into the pitch, turning their body toward it. When they do this, their weight shifts to their back foot. Then they shift their weight forward and swing the bat across the plate. Both of these batters take less than *one-fifth of a second* to complete this move.

There are two parts to a baseball swing. The first one-tenth of a second is when the batter swings the bat. The second one-tenth of a second is the reaction of the bat. A hitter like Davis swings the bat with a force of about 50 pounds. As the bat moves into part two of the swing, the force on the batter's hands and arms increases about five times. The bat is moving at about 70 mph at this point in the swing.

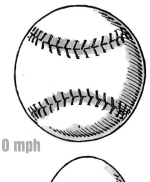

0 mph

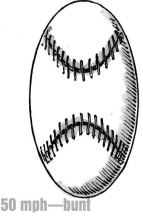

50 mph—bunt

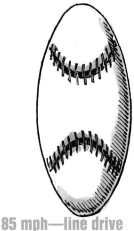

85 mph—line drive

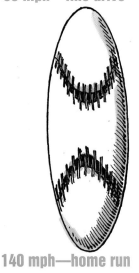

140 mph—home run

Bats Meets Ball

The bat and ball collision takes about *1/1000th of a second*. The tremendous impact of the pitched ball meeting a swinging bat squishes the ball to about half its original diameter. Like a spring, all that wound yarn squeezes together and then recoils as the ball flies off the bat, sending it toward the outer reaches of the ballpark. It comes back down to earth only when the gravity overcomes the force.

When the ball comes off the bat, there's usually a lot of spin. If Eric Davis were to jump on a pitch and pull the ball down the left field line, the ball would be spinning counterclockwise at the rate of about 2,000 rpm. If he were to hit the ball just below its center, the fly ball that would result would have backspin. And if he were to be fooled by a dropping curveball and hit the ball above center, the ground ball would move with topspin.

Because of the counterclockwise spin, a ball hit to left field by a right-handed hitter will normally hook or curve toward the left field foul line. The spin causes the air pressure on the left side of the ball to be less than the air pressure on the right. More air pressure on the right pushes the ball to the left. A ball hit to right field by a left-handed hitter will usually hook toward the right field foul line. A ball hit on the button, with little spin, will usually head toward center field.

A ball must be hit so that it travels at a minimum of a 35-degree angle to send it over the fence. Eric Davis (the right-handed

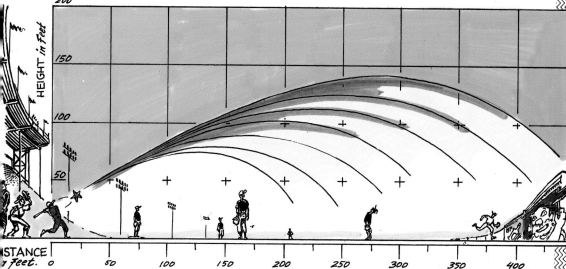

home run hitter) swings the bat with more of an upward angle than Tony Gwynn (the left-handed line drive hitter). Gwynn is more intent on hitting the ball on the line, taking a level swing, with the bat hitting the ball just in front of the plate. If his timing is slightly off, he can still get a hit. If he swings the bat a fraction of a second early, he will line the ball between first and second. A fraction of a second late, and he will line the ball to left field. If he were to swing and hit just underneath the ball, he might hit a high line drive in the right-center gap; a little on top of the ball, he will hit a ground ball that will go through the infield.

Because of the angle of his swing, Gwynn will hit far fewer home runs as well as fewer pop-ups. But if Eric Davis miscalculates the timing of his swing using his slight uppercut, he will tend to either top the ball and ground out if he swings early or hit under the ball and pop up to an infielder if he swings late.

Both men hit the ball with the same amount of force. One hits for average, and one hits for home runs; both are considered hitting stars of the game.

As Hall of Fame pitcher Warren Spahn said, "Hitting is timing. Pitching is upsetting that timing." What Spahn didn't say is that pitching is also knowing how to use the principles of aerodynamics so that the ball travels to the plate the way the pitcher intended.

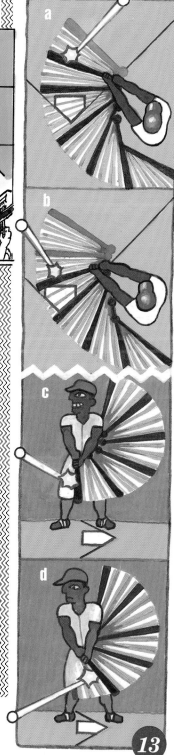

Hitting is timing: a) an early swing by a line drive hitter; b) a late swing by a line frive hitter; c) an early swing by a home run hitter; and d) a late swing by a home run hitter

13

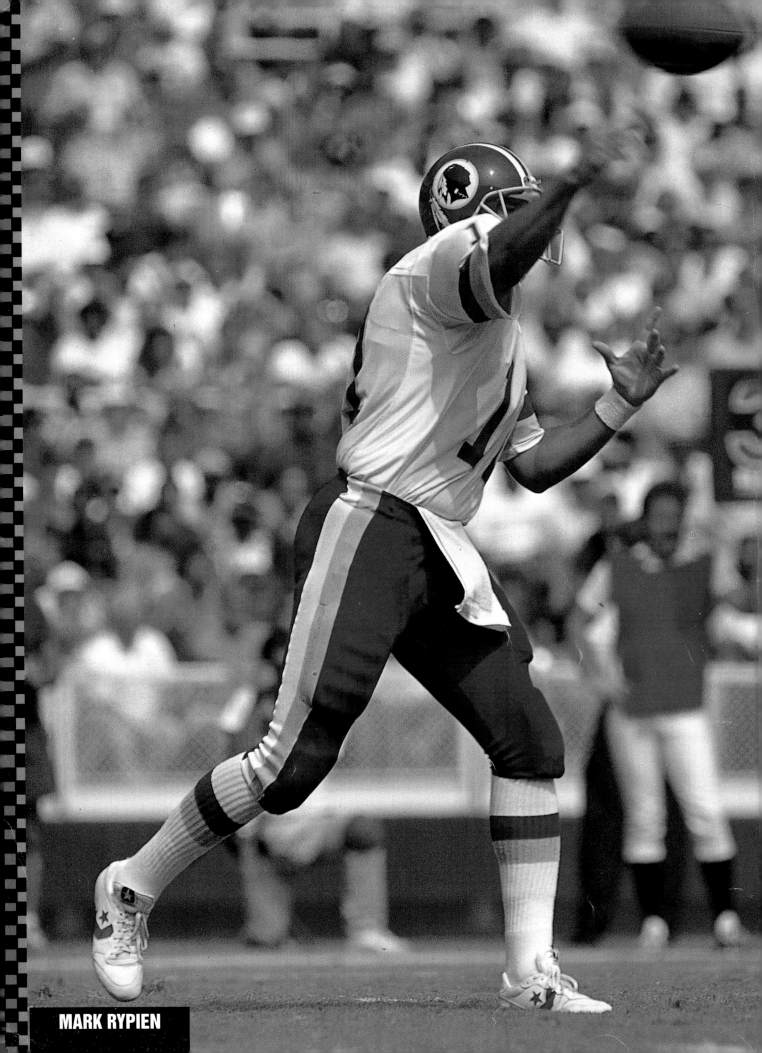

MARK RYPIEN

THROWING A PERFECT SPIRAL

"Mark Rypien fades back behind a wall of protection and lofts a perfect spiral pass 40 yards downfield into the outstretched arms of Art Monk for a touchdown."

Football has come a long way since it was first played in 1874. At that time, Harvard University played a game known as Boston football, similar to today's soccer. They invited a rugby team from McGill University in Canada to come and play one game of Boston football and one game of rugby. The Harvard players loved rugby, which had been developed in England by a frustrated soccer player who wanted to carry the ball instead of kick it. The Harvard players combined rugby with their own form of soccer and gave birth to American football.

The ball used in the new game took the basic shape of the rugby ball, because it was easier to carry. Today's professional football, though smaller and less round, still looks much like the ball used in that first football game.

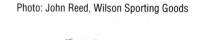

Photo: John Reed, Wilson Sporting Goods

According to the official rules of the National Football League, the football is to be an inflated (12½ to 13½ pounds per square inch) rubber bladder enclosed in a pebble-grained, leather case (natural tan color) without grooves or folds of any kind. Its shape is called a prolate spheroid—the oblong shape you know so well—and it must weigh between 14 and 15 ounces. This is an odd ball.

The football was originally designed only to be carried or kicked. But it took on a new function with the legalization of the forward pass in 1906. This change also introduced some new and different aerodynamic considerations into the game.

Just as the earth spins on its axis, that imaginary line drawn through the center of an object around which it rotates, so does a football. But a football has more than one axis. It has a long axis, along the length of the ball, and it has a short axis, through the middle of the ball. The direction the football is facing greatly affects the aerodynamics. Is the ball traveling point first, as when it is passed? Or side first, as during a kickoff? This is called *orientation*. Earlier, we learned that the direction a baseball's stitches face affects the ball's aerodynamics, but in football, the orientation affects the ball even more.

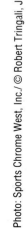

Photo: Sports Chrome West, Inc./ © Robert Tringali, Jr.

15

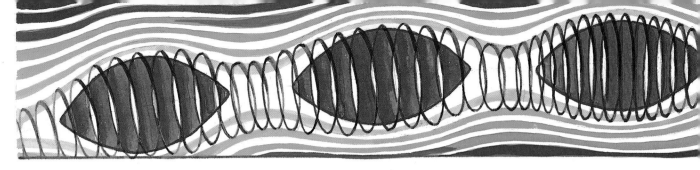

Faster:
Less air resistance

THE SPIRAL PASS

The pass of least air resistance in football is the perfect spiral pass, in which the ball spins around its long axis. If a right-handed quarterback throws the ball, the spin from the receiver's viewpoint goes counterclockwise. A left-handed QB, like Boomer Esiason, throws the ball so that from his receiver's viewpoint the football is spinning clockwise. This spin and the ball's orientation and speed (about 50 mph) allow it to travel through the air with its nose leading the way. In this direction, the air hits the smallest amount of its surface, so there is the the least amount of drag.

The tight spin of a spiral pass breaks up the air molecules. And, as we've already found out, choppy air means less air resistance. So the ball's direction remains the same throughout its flight.

To ensure that a pass spirals down field accurately and with the greatest distance, a quarterback must grip the ball on its side. Unfortunately, this side grip doesn't allow a quarterback to apply as much force as a baseball player can to get the ball downfield. So a quarterback must use spin to compensate for lack of speed. This turns the ball into something of a gyroscope, spinning around its long axis. A spiral pass spins about 10 revolutions per second.

If the ball is misthrown, it will wobble. Wobbling means more of the ball's surface is exposed to the passing air molecules, which means there's more drag on the ball and it's slowed down considerably. Defensive backs like Ronnie Lott gobble up these wobbly, shortened passes, intercepting and returning them for big yards. Lott makes his living partly because of these increased aerodynamic forces on the ball.

JUST FOR KICKS

There are two other ways a football can move through the air. One of them is seen on a kickoff. Using a running start, a kicker hits the ball with his foot below the centerpoint of the ball. The ball then sails end-over-end in the direction it has been kicked.

As long as the ball is in the air and is not affected by wind gusts that could twist its path, it will travel in the direction it was kicked. Because of its tumbling motion, there is unequal air pressure around the ball. The side facing the airstream has more pressure, so with the tumble of the ball, the pressure is constantly changing from side to side. This unequal aerodynamic force means that a kickoff traveling at the same speed as a spiral pass will meet an air resistance nearly 10 times stronger.

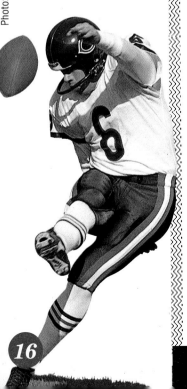

KEVIN BUTLER

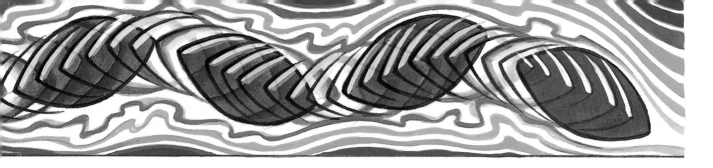

The reason a kicker can kick a ball so much farther than a quarterback can pass the ball is that leg muscles are much stronger than arm muscles. The kicker also has a running start and can increase the speed of the ball to overcome the air resistance. A professional kicker can kick a ball close to 80 mph. A typical spiral pass only reaches a speed of about 50 mph.

The third way a football moves through the air is when it is punted. To get the most distance, a punter must learn to punt the ball in a spiral motion. But in punting, distance is not the only factor that must be taken into consideration. "Hang time," or the time the ball is in the air, is also critical to allow tacklers to get downfield to stop the punt receiver.

A punter has to calculate the angle at which the ball is kicked. The greater the angle, the higher the ball will go, and the longer the ball will remain in the air. Unfortunately, kicking the ball higher means that it won't travel as far. On average, the angle for punting a football that will deliver the best combination of distance and hang time falls somewhere between 40 and 60 degrees.

Punting a spiral is much more difficult than passing a spiral. A right-footed punter must angle his leg from right to left as he kicks underneath the ball. As the ball spirals upward, it looks very much like a spiral pass. But once the punt passes the top point of its flight path and starts to fall, the air pressure changes. The reason is the ball has lost a lot of its speed. At this point, the ball is almost broadside as it begins its downward descent. More of the football's surface is getting bombarded by air molecules. This creates added air pressure that twists the ball and makes it tumble as it falls.

Because of its shape, a football is subject to the whim of the winds. The slightest twist or turn in a quarterback's delivery might send the ball on a path of great aerodynamic resistance—and right into the hands of a defender.

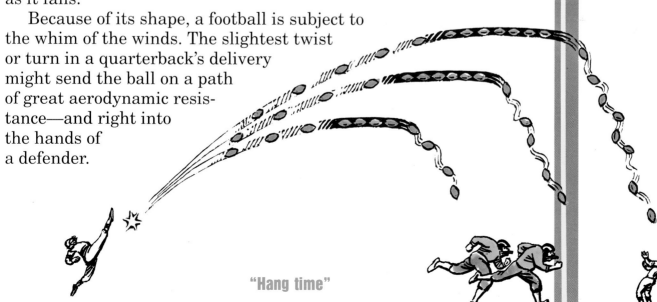

"Hang time"

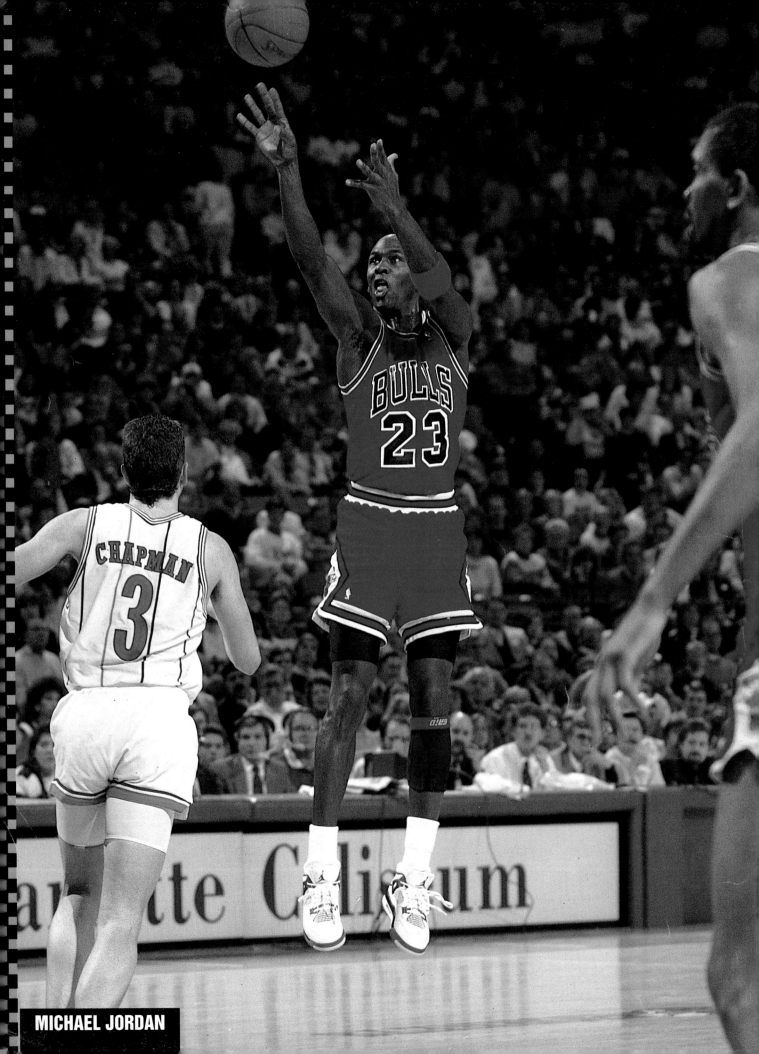

MICHAEL JORDAN

JUMP SHOTS AND BACKBOARDS

"T he Pistons lead the Bulls by 2 with seven seconds to go. The ball is inbounded to Paxson under the basket. Paxson feeds the ball to Michael Jordan. Jordan is in the front court, with three seconds on the clock. Jordan dribbles left, just beyond the three-point line, and from 25 feet he fires. It's nothing but net as the buzzer sounds, and the Bulls down the Pistons by 1."

Little in sports compares with the excitement of the last two minutes of a close professional basketball game. But how do those guys do it? How do they seem to know exactly how to release the ball at the right height, at the right speed, and with the right trajectory so that it touches nothing but net?

They do it by applying spin to the ball and by practicing the release of the ball at many different angles and heights. Of course, it's important to have a "feel" for the speed necessary to project the ball toward the center of the basket so the aerodynamics it encounters doesn't make the shot short.

The official basketball is about 9½ inches in diameter (about 30 inches around) and weighs 20 to 22 ounces. When it's dropped from a height of 6 feet, the ball will bounce as high as 54 inches. Like a football, it has a pebbled surface designed primarily for grip. The basket is 18 inches in diameter, so the ball is just a little larger than half the size of the basket. A standard backboard is 6 feet by 4 feet, and the top of the backboard is 40 inches above the top of the rim. The rim is set 10 feet above the playing surface.

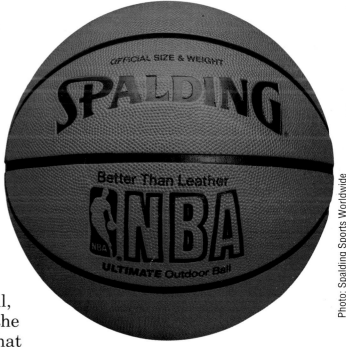

HITTING A SHOT

In talking about the aerodynamics of basketball, we are basically describing the jump shot and the free throw. There are few aerodynamic forces that affect a slam dunk or a lay-in. And the aerodynamics of a shot bounced off the backboard are much the same as the aerodynamics of a jump shot aimed at the center of the rim.

The main ingredients of a successful basketball shot are spin, angle of release, and speed. One of the basics of basketball is that a successful shot is pushed by a player's fingertips rather than by

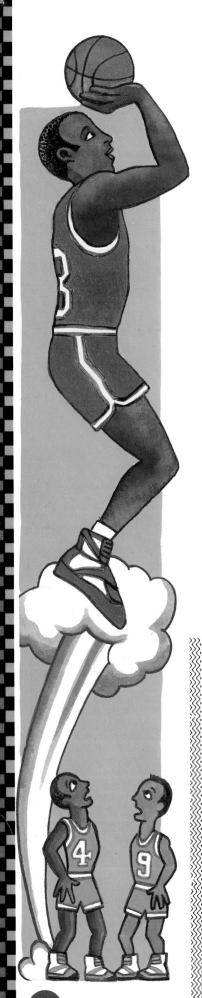

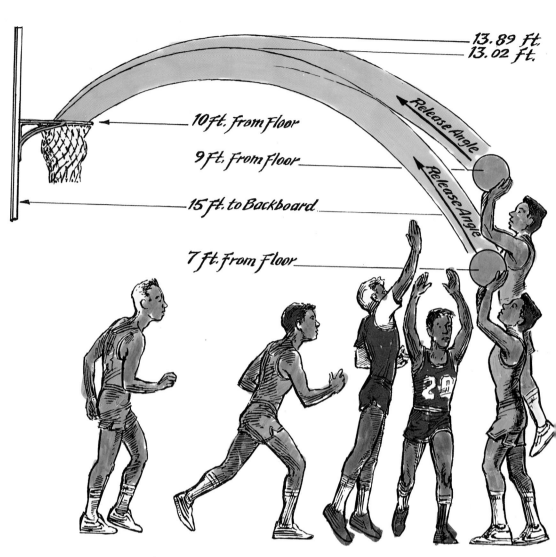

13.89 Ft.
13.02 Ft.

Release Angle

Release Angle

10 ft. from Floor

9 ft. from Floor

15 ft. to Backboard

7 ft. from Floor

the palm of the hand. This gives the shooter better control and, by releasing the ball with a flick of the wrist, allows him to put backspin on it.

When a basketball with backspin hits the rim or the ground, it loses its speed, spin, and energy faster than one with forward spin or no spin. This is important, because a ball shot with backspin doesn't bounce wildly off the backboard or rim; it sort of "dies" on the backboard, giving it a much better chance of falling through the rim. Arnold "Red" Auerbach, former coach of the Boston Celtics and one of the greatest basketball coaches around, says that backspin "helps the ball to be 'lucky.'" From a physics perspective, luck has nothing to do with it.

Typically, a basketball shot taken from 25 feet or less is in the air less than one second. This is fortunate for the last-second heroics of Jordan, Thomas, Bird, Mullens, and friends. The speed of the ball is also pretty slow, when compared to a baseball. A basketball in flight averages about 20 to 30 feet per second. Despite this, air resistance plays a part in netting a jump shot.

ANGLE OF ATTACK

For the ball to clear the rim and go through the hoop, it cannot be shot at an angle of less than 32 degrees. If you think of 90 degrees as being straight up, then 32 degrees is about a third of the way up. The most successful angle for a shot 10 to 25 feet from the basket is between 40 and 50 degrees.

Most basketball players release the ball about 1 to 2 feet above their heads. Since most basketball players are well over 6 feet tall, above their heads is somewhere between 7 and 9 feet from the floor. The best percentage shot for making a basket is with a higher arch. There are two reasons: a higher angle will arc over a taller player, and a higher angle gives a better trajectory toward the basket.

The air resistance a basketball meets is not just a lot of hot air. Let's return to spin on the ball. A basketball with backspin (see Baseball) meets less air resistance than a ball shot without spin. If you shoot a spinning ball and a nonspinning ball with the same angle and the same speed, the nonspinning ball will fall shorter than the backspinning ball.

But a basketball with backspin does encounter some air resistance. If the drag on the ball isn't figured into a jump shot, the ball would fall about a foot short of its mark. To compensate for this drag, a player must increase the speed of the shot by about 5 percent. The longer the ball is in the air, the greater the air resistance it encounters. So Clyde Drexler has to shoot the ball with even greater speed and a larger margin of error if he wants to sink a desperation shot from half court. Air resistance also changes the flight of the ball: the angle that the ball falls is steeper than its path upward. This effect also increases the difficulty of Drexler's long shot, because it narrows the path through which the ball can successfully fly toward the basket.

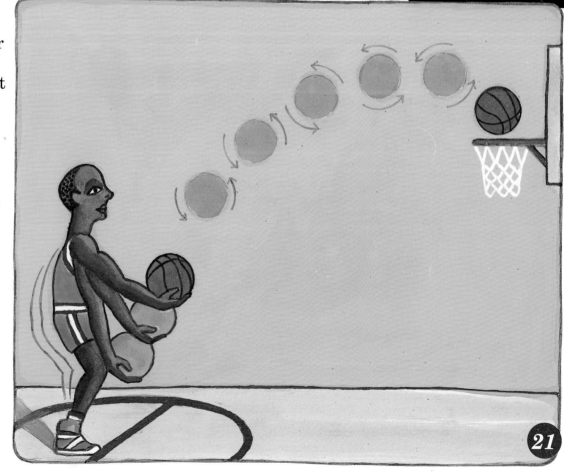

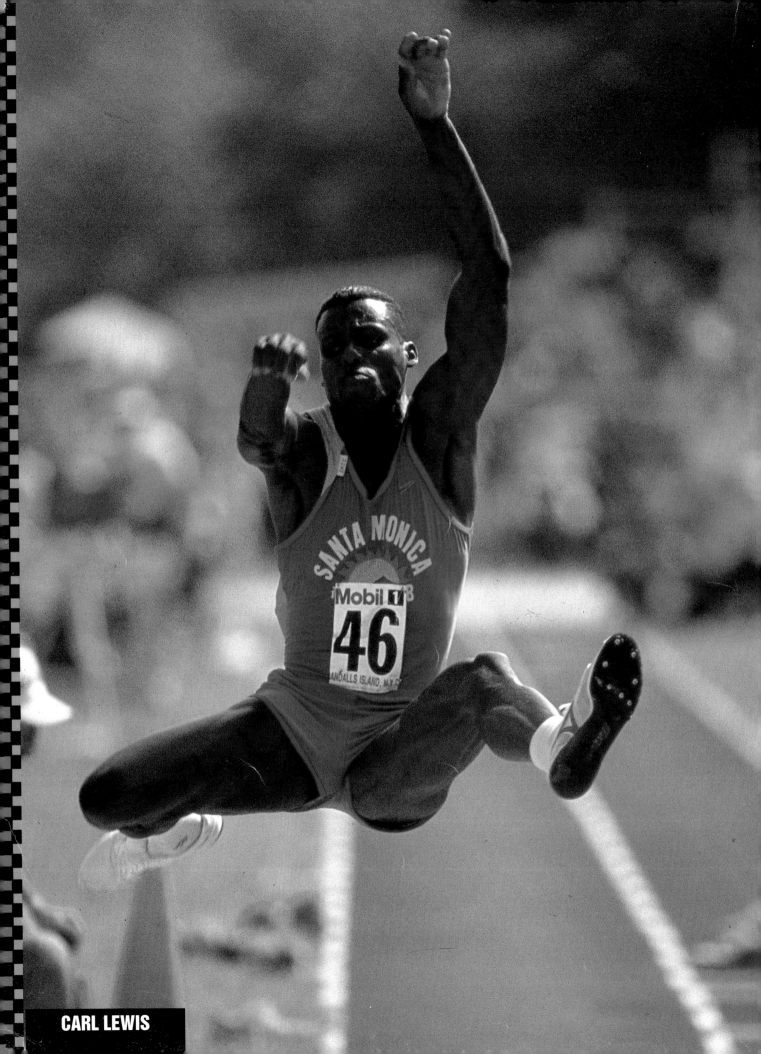

CARL LEWIS

TAKING OFF WITH TRACK AND FIELD

Is Carl Lewis the most aerodynamically designed human? You might think so, since he runs faster and jumps farther than most other humans. But he and other track and field athletes encounter the forces of air resistance and drag.

The 1968 Olympic Games in Mexico City show us how powerful the aerodynamic forces are. The altitude there is over a mile above sea level. As we go higher, air molecules are less crammed together, or less dense. Since they are less dense, there is less air resistance and less drag holding the runners back. Runners ran a little over 2 percent faster there than at sea level. World records were set at the Mexico City games in the 100-, 200-, 400-, and 800-meter runs and in the pole vault, long jump, and triple jump.

Up until now, we have been talking about the effects of aerodynamics on balls that have been thrown, kicked, or hit. In the language of physics, these balls traveling through the air are considered projectiles. In the sprint, the long jump, the pole vault, and the high jump, human bodies are the projectiles, the objects hurled through the air.

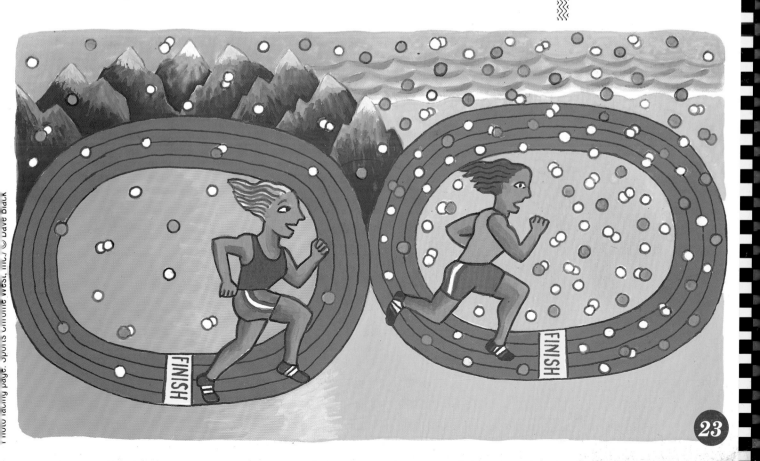

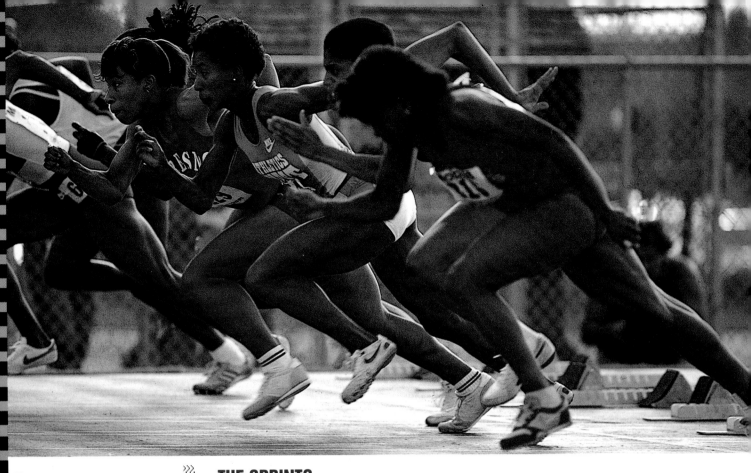

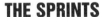

Photos: Sports Chrome West, Inc./ © Mitchell B. Reibel

THE SPRINTS

Runners to your mark. Get set. GO! Although we don't usually think about it this way, our legs actually lose energy when we run. They have to lift our bodies and speed up and slow down, and our feet keep hitting the ground. Runners have to overcome this energy loss. In addition, runners' legs have to battle the forces of air resistance and drag beating against their chest as they try to outpace their opponents.

When runners sprint without the aid of any wind, they lose about 10 percent of their power to the forces of drag. In a 100-meter race, this could mean as much as a one-second difference. If runners could cut one second off their 100-meter times, they would be running 100 meters in less than 9 seconds. The current world record, without the benefit of wind, is 9.86 seconds. It's held by Carl Lewis.

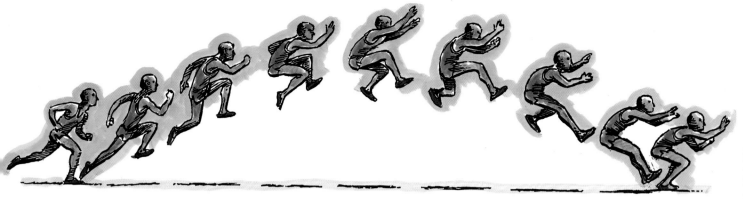

THE LONG JUMP

Carl Lewis may not hold the long jump record now, but many track watchers expect that if anyone can travel over 30 feet in the air, it will be Lewis. So let's look at Carl Lewis as projectile.

In the long jump, Lewis runs as fast as he can toward the take-off line. He jumps, raising his body as high as possible, and then as he is falling back to earth, he bends his knees, landing at the end of the sand pit. One problem all long jumpers face is that humans are not great jumpers. For example, only half the energy Lewis builds up running carries him during his leap. For Lewis to reach a world record in the long jump, he has to leap just over 3 feet high as he takes off. He stays in the air only about one second.

The air resistance Lewis feels starts as he is running toward the takeoff line. It slows his speed as he heads down the lane. After he is airborne, the drag effect on Lewis's body reduces the distance of his jump by almost 7 inches.

If he were to long jump in Mexico City, he could reduce that 7-inch drag force by about 25 percent, because of the thinner air. That would add almost 2 inches to his leap. In fact, this was how Bob Beamon was able to leap 29 feet 2 inches. Lewis has since leaped three-fourths of an inch farther (a lot in a sport like the long jump), but that took place on the same day that Mike Powell jumped 29 feet 4½ inches.

We don't know how long these records will stand. But former world record holder Beamon suggests that because of his speed, Lewis will be the first to crash through the aerodynamic barrier of 30 feet.

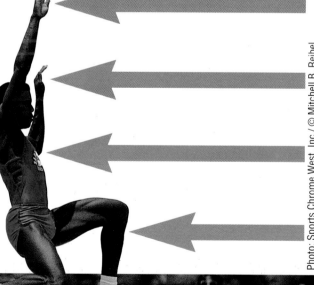

CARL LEWIS

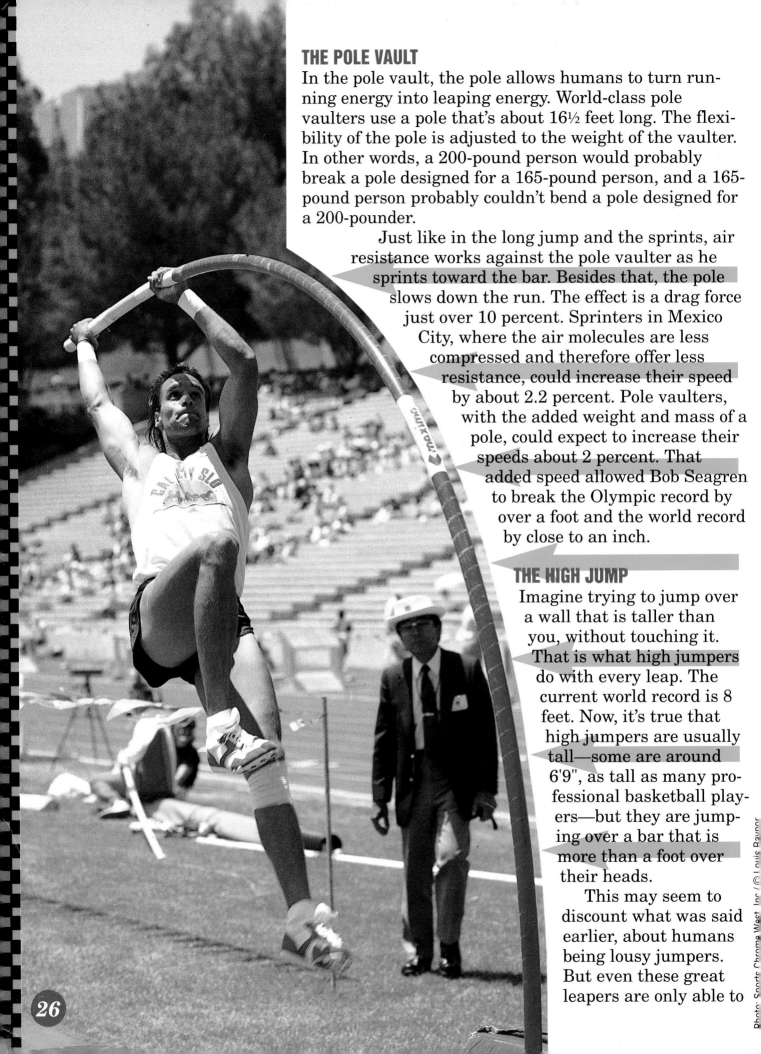

THE POLE VAULT

In the pole vault, the pole allows humans to turn running energy into leaping energy. World-class pole vaulters use a pole that's about 16½ feet long. The flexibility of the pole is adjusted to the weight of the vaulter. In other words, a 200-pound person would probably break a pole designed for a 165-pound person, and a 165-pound person probably couldn't bend a pole designed for a 200-pounder.

Just like in the long jump and the sprints, air resistance works against the pole vaulter as he sprints toward the bar. Besides that, the pole slows down the run. The effect is a drag force just over 10 percent. Sprinters in Mexico City, where the air molecules are less compressed and therefore offer less resistance, could increase their speed by about 2.2 percent. Pole vaulters, with the added weight and mass of a pole, could expect to increase their speeds about 2 percent. That added speed allowed Bob Seagren to break the Olympic record by over a foot and the world record by close to an inch.

THE HIGH JUMP

Imagine trying to jump over a wall that is taller than you, without touching it. That is what high jumpers do with every leap. The current world record is 8 feet. Now, it's true that high jumpers are usually tall—some are around 6'9", as tall as many professional basketball players—but they are jumping over a bar that is more than a foot over their heads.

This may seem to discount what was said earlier, about humans being lousy jumpers. But even these great leapers are only able to convert half of the energy of their 100-foot, J-shaped running approach into a leap. They start this approach about 10 to 18 feet out from the bar and 100 feet back, curving toward it for the leap. World-class jumpers make this approach in only 17 strides.

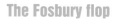

Photo: Sports Chrome West, Inc./ © Robert Tringali, Jr.

The Fosbury flop

The J-shape approach is to accommodate one of the major changes in high jumping. In 1968, Richard Fosbury added 2½ inches to the world record high jump by flopping over the bar backward, rather than using the conventional straddle approach. It shocked the track and field world and changed high jumping forever.

The Fosbury flop, as it is now known, lets the high jumper take off with a much higher angle than the straddle leap. This happens because the leap places the jumper's center of gravity, or weight, directly over the launching foot. This allows for a much better distribution of the leaper's weight than with the straddle. In addition to the improved center of gravity, the flop lets a jumper get his or her hips high over the bar so they don't hit it as they complete the jump.

Air resistance works against the jumper at every step and leap. The first part of the body over the bar is the head, which breaks up the airflow and creates less air resistance for the rest of the body. The jumper holds his arms close to his sides, and he brings his legs over last.

In the straddle approach, the jumper's legs are spread apart. One leg goes over the bar first, followed by the second leg and body. The jumper's arms are spread. These flailing arms and legs increase the air resistance and the drag on the body.

But like a football cutting nose first through the air, the Fosbury flop provides a better aerodynamic approach. Fosbury went to the drawing board, like a car designer trying to create a more aerodynamic shape for better gas mileage, and in the process redesigned high jumping. By cutting down on the drag and increasing his liftoff angle, Fosbury set a new standard for the study of man in flight. What other sports could be improved by somehow changing the aerodynamics involved? If you can figure that out, who knows, you might be the next Fosbury, or the next world record holder.

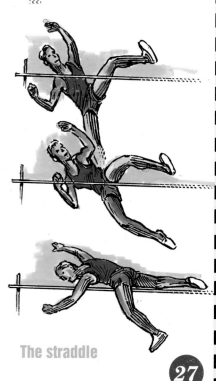

The straddle

GOLF'S HOOKS AND SLICES

"**B**etsy King steps up to the tee. The crowd behind her hushes as she prepares to hit her drive. She brings her wood back, and with a stroke as smooth as silk, she drives her golf ball down the center of the fairway, over 230 yards from the tee. She's in perfect position to chip to the green."

If you have ever picked up a golf club and tried to hit that tiny white dimpled ball, you know that golf is one of the most difficult and frustrating games being played today. There are so many different factors that can affect the flight of the ball. Only some of them are aerodynamically related.

The game begins simply enough by placing a golf ball on a tee. That's the easy part. Before we bring our club down on that teed-up ball, it might be helpful to take a closer look at the ball itself. It has gone through numerous changes in its history.

A LITTLE HISTORY

For over 150 years, the golf ball actually consisted of a piece of stitched cowhide filled with boiled feathers. Called the featherie, and based on a Roman design, it was said to have refined the game of golf with its superior flight characteristics.

Golfers then began to use the Gutta-percha ball. It was first produced in St. Andrews, Scotland, home of the British Open golf tournament. This was the precursor to our modern ball, made from a substance like East Indian rubber that hardened when it was exposed to air. As we will explain shortly, this ball was originally covered with nicks to help it stay aloft. The nicks were later replaced by molded dimples. These dimples marked the first major aerodynamic change in golf.

Today's official ball cannot weigh more than 1.62 ounces and cannot have a diameter of less than 1.68 inches. The ball must be spherical in shape. And, no matter which way you hook or slice it, a golf ball has to be the same through and through,

MEG MALLON

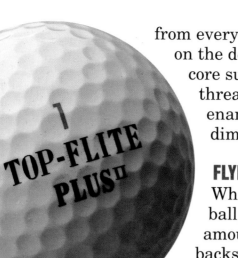

from every angle. The ball is built on the design of a solid rubber core surrounded by rubber thread, covered with a hard enamel and, of course, its dimpled coating.

FLYING DIMPLES

When a golf club hits a golf ball, it causes an incredible amount of backspin. The backspin together with the dimples give a golf ball its lift. If a ball were hit without backspin, it would encounter greater air resistance and would not stay in the air as long. Adding thousands of rpm of spin breaks up the air and can add a couple of extra seconds of flight time to a drive. That couple of seconds can translate into 80 to 100 yards in added distance.

The golf ball's dimples serve the same function as a baseball's stitches. They catch the air traveling around the ball. Since the ball has a backspin, the air on the top of the ball is moving faster because it is traveling with the airstream, and the air underneath is traveling slower because it is moving *into* the airstream. The air circling around a backspinning golf ball creates less pressure on the top of the ball and greater pressure underneath it. This difference in air speed and pressure creates a golf ball's lift. Without the dimples to catch the air, a golf ball would only travel about one-fourth as far.

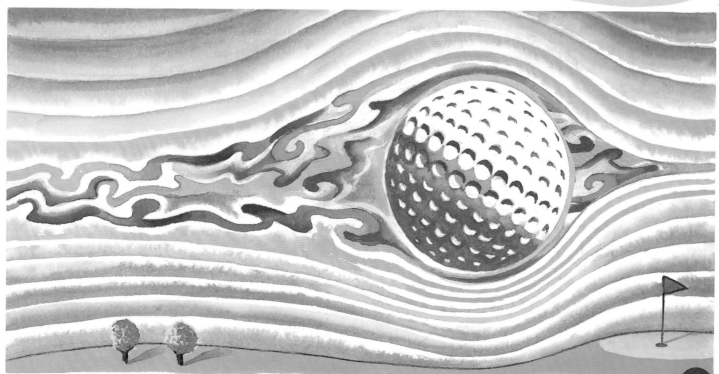

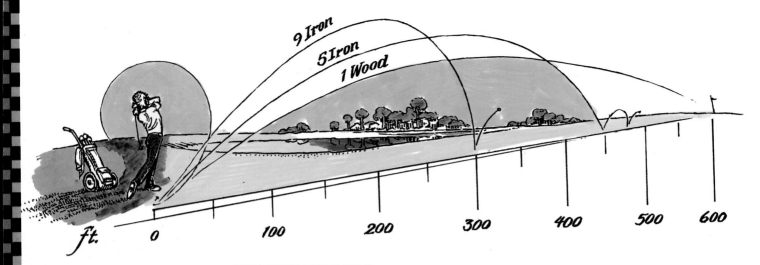

THE DRIVE FOR PAR

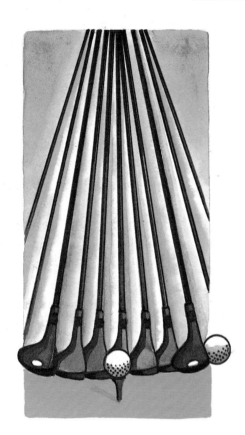

The collision between club and ball lasts for about 1/2000th of a second. It is amazing how much can go wrong in that short blink of an eye. If the ball is struck with the front of the club, it will be sent spinning clockwise and slice off to the right. If the ball is hit with the back of the club, it will spin counterclockwise and hook off to the left. Because of the short time the ball is in contact with the club, there is no way to correct a ball that has been hit wrong. Once it is hit, all the golfer can do is watch.

As the golf ball lifts off the tee, it is traveling about 250 feet per second. The golf ball immediately encounters the effects of lift, air resistance and drag, and gravity. In its first stage of flight, lift actually allows a golf ball to overcome the effects of gravity, keeping it airborne longer than if it weren't spinning. A golf ball's flight can also be affected by temperature, altitude, humidity, winds, trees, birds, and other golfers standing in the way. FORE! But the primary factors at work are lift, because of the backspin on the ball, drag, because of air resistance acting against the motion of the ball, and gravity, which forces the ball downward.

THE CLUBS

The clubs also have a lot to do with golf's aerodynamics. There are two kinds of clubs, woods and irons. The woods are for driving the ball long distances. They have large blocklike heads, traditionally made of wood. The irons and the wedges are for hitting and chipping the ball shorter distances. They are made of metal, with narrower heads. There is also a putter, but since the ball is already on the ground when this club is used, there are no aerodynamics associated with it.

Golf club faces have a slight angle. This allows the club to hit under the ball and apply backspin. The greater the angle, the higher the ball travels. The higher the ball goes up, the shorter the distance it travels. Spin allows a player to get greater lift and a higher trajectory on the ball. The ball spins about 8,000 rpm when hit with an iron and 3,000 rpm when hit with a wood.

As the golf ball clears the tee, its flight path is fairly straight, with just a slight rise. But as the ball begins to lose speed, the effects of lift, spin, and drag all decrease, and the ball falls under the control of gravity and begins its rather steep fall to earth. On a tee shot, the best angle to achieve the longest time in the air is about 20 degrees. A higher trajectory will mean that most of the speed will be used to lift the ball higher rather than carry it farther. When the speed is lost, gravity once again takes over and pulls the ball down. With the more lofted angle of the irons, the idea is to hit the ball a shorter distance, so a higher and shorter trajectory, with greater backspin, is best.

The trick to hitting a golf ball is learning how to use the aerodynamics of the ball to your advantage. This requires hitting with the center portion of the club head, not lifting the head, not hitting it with the front or back of the club, not misdirecting your feet, and not yanking the club too fast through the swing and turning the club head. Hitting a golf ball hard does not always get the best aerodynamic results. Hitting the ball correctly will.

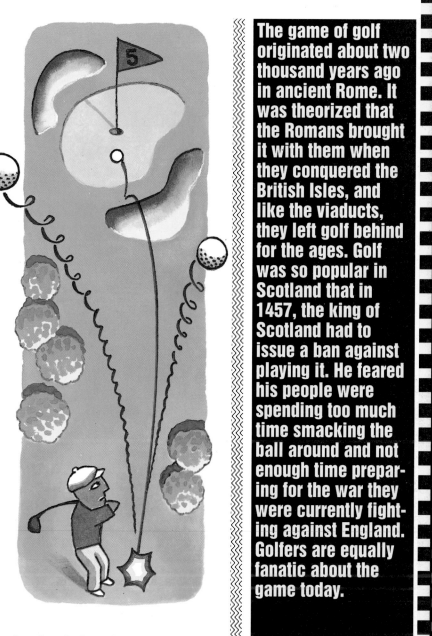

The game of golf originated about two thousand years ago in ancient Rome. It was theorized that the Romans brought it with them when they conquered the British Isles, and like the viaducts, they left golf behind for the ages. Golf was so popular in Scotland that in 1457, the king of Scotland had to issue a ban against playing it. He feared his people were spending too much time smacking the ball around and not enough time preparing for the war they were currently fighting against England. Golfers are equally fanatic about the game today.

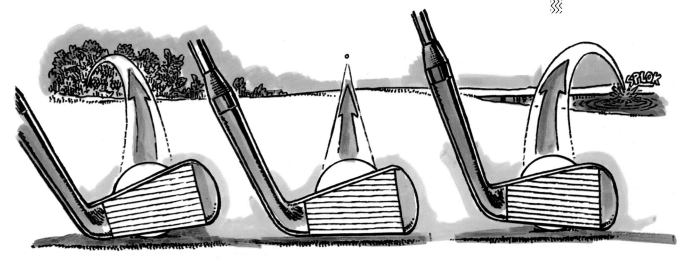

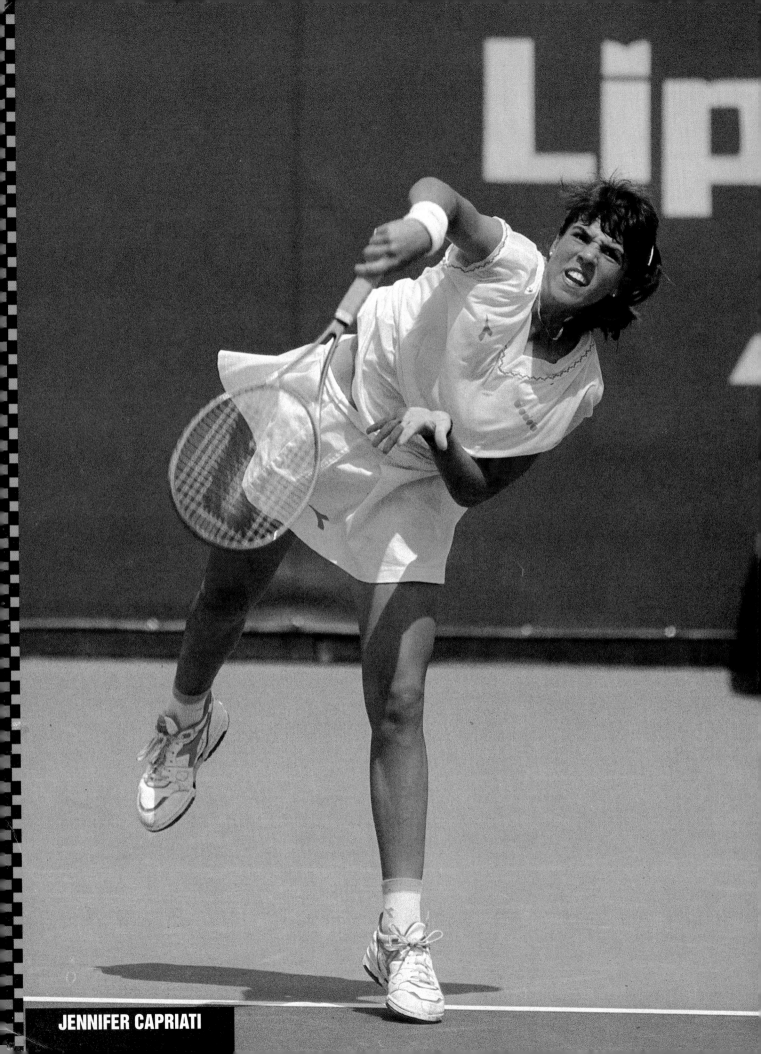

JENNIFER CAPRIATI

WHY TENNIS BALLS ARE FUZZY

"**M**onica Seles tosses the ball up and with a grunt, serves a hard topspin smash to Gabriela Sabatini. The bright fluorescent yellow ball hits the hard court surface just in front of the service line and suddenly kicks off to the right. Sabatini lunges to return the serve. Seles takes the short return to her forehand, and with the racket at its lowest point on her backswing, she brings the racket through with a great grunt and crushes a topspin forehand winner down the right side of the court."

Tennis is a game of spin, angle, and aerodynamic manipulations. Like golf and baseball, tennis is about hitting a ball with an instrument, in this case, the strings of a racket. And like golf, the aerodynamics of the game involve the ball in flight, after it has been hit. In tennis, one of the most important features affecting aerodynamics is the fuzz on the ball.

A tennis ball is a hollow rubber sphere that is pumped up to a high inner air pressure and then covered with rough felt. It weighs about 2 ounces, measures about 2 inches in diameter, and has two indented seams. Like a golf ball's dimples, these seams allow air to pass around the ball and improve lift.

FUZZY ACTION

Since the most common shot in tennis is the topspin, the fuzz acts to break up the air, so the ball meets less air resistance. The fuzz also allows the ball to stay momentarily on the racket so the player can apply spin. The racket starts back low and moves toward the ball. And the racket face is usually slightly angled, too. When Seles makes contact with the ball, she gives it an upward force that causes a topspin motion.

MONICA SELES

33

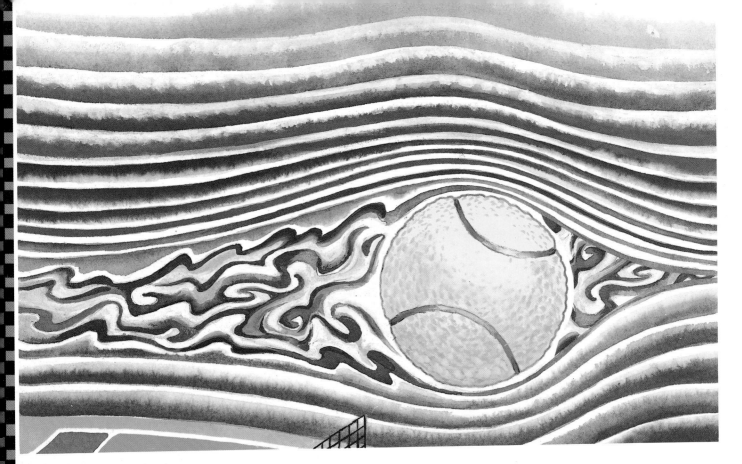

The air underneath the ball is picked up by the fuzz, causing it to move faster than the air on top of the ball. The bottom of the ball is moving with the airstream. The top of the ball is moving against the airstream. This action creates less air pressure underneath the ball and greater air pressure on top of the ball, which helps push it down. Topspin helps keep hard hit balls on the court. It also makes the ball move faster after it bounces.

The fuzz also increases the drag on the ball. This is why Martina Navratilova can hit the ball as hard as she does, at the height and trajectory she does, without sending it flying off the court. Drag changes the flight of the shot from a smooth curve and forces the ball down at a steeper angle. If the ball were smooth, it would not be able to catch the air around it and create the same downward effects of a topspin hit.

In play, some tennis balls that have lost their fuzz actually become livelier, and they bounce more. But they lose a great deal of their aerodynamic spinning effect.

A second kind of tennis swing is a backhand chip shot. Because many players lack the strength of Navratilova or Seles to power a backhand shot with topspin (which is why there are now many two-handed backhand hitters), they use the backhand chip shot. A player starts his or her racket high and brings it down alongside the ball, putting a backspin on it. This shot carries deeper into the court but at a much slower speed than a topspin shot (if it were hit too hard, it would simply fly off the court).

POWER SERVES

The final shot affected by the forces of aerodynamics is the serve. A player like Steffi Graf might use a big twist serve. In this case, the ball is hit on the top and side. This creates some topspin but also gives the ball a sideways spin, which makes it curve to either the right or left depending on which side was struck. This added spin angle changes the air pressure on the sides of the ball. On a ball curving toward the left side of the court, the air pressure is greater on the right side than on the left. On a ball curving toward the right side, the air pressure is greater on the left.

Though there are other forces at work in tennis, none would matter without the proper aerodynamics of that fuzzy ball being bashed about. What happens when the ball hits the ground is entirely determined by what happens while the ball is in flight. Just ask anyone who has been on the other side of Graf's forehand smash.

Photo: Sports Chrome West, Inc./ © Louis Raynor

MARTINA NAVRATILOVA

THE SWEET SPOT OF A TENNIS RACKET

The sweet spot of a tennis racket is that part of the racket face that returns the ball most powerfully and with the least vibration. On the rackets of just a few years ago, the sweet spot was located a couple of inches above the base of the racket face. Today's larger faced rackets have increased the size of the sweet spot 300 percent. It now extends in an ellipse (an elongated oval) toward the top of the racket face.

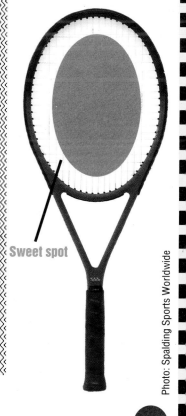

Sweet spot

Photo: Spalding Sports Worldwide

35

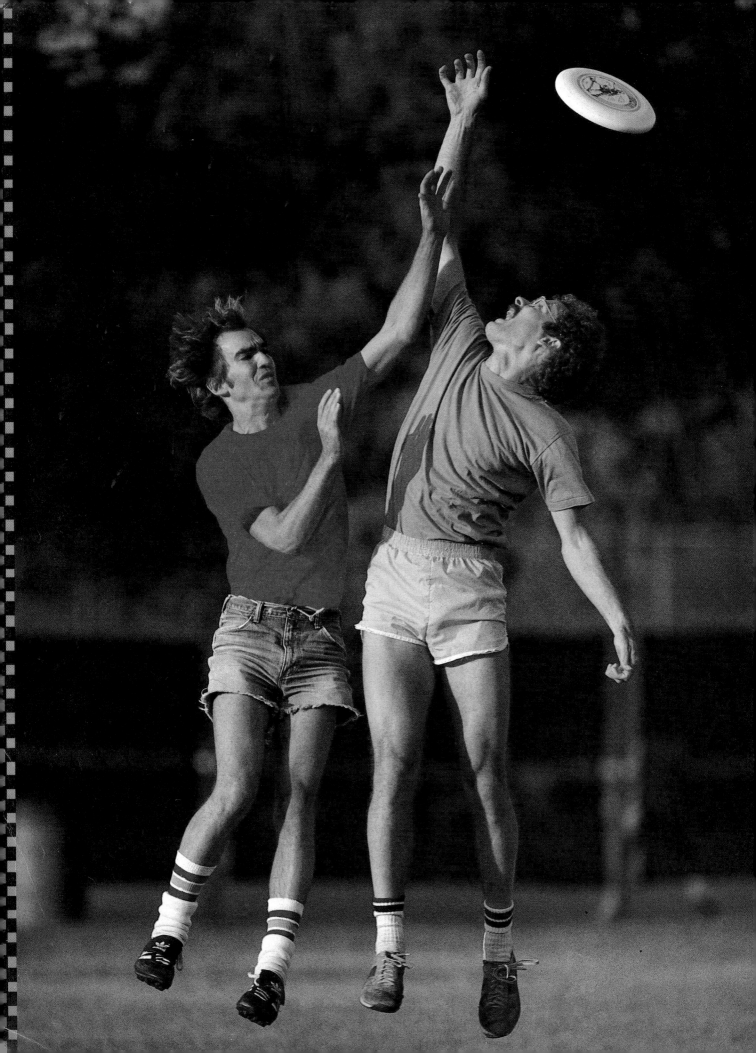

OF FLYING PLASTIC AND DOGS

When Fred Morrison, the father of the Frisbee, first sold his "Pluto Platter," as the Frisbee was called then, he told people that even though the plate seemed to fly on its own, it really rode along an invisible wire. Morrison sold the invisible wire for one cent a foot and threw in the Pluto Platter for free with every hundred feet of invisible wire purchased.

The design of the Frisbee hasn't changed much since Morrison sold his idea to the Wham-O Corporation in 1957. Wham-O does not include any pieces of invisible string, but the Frisbee certainly does fly. How it flies is a story of aerodynamics.

Whether soaring, curving, diving, hovering, or returning like a boomerang, the Frisbee is being pushed and guided through the air by air pressure, lift, and drag. The air resistance the Frisbee meets in flight slows down its rate of spin, its speed, its motion, and its fall to earth. It also causes the Frisbee to float just before it is caught or hits the ground. This floating is caused by the slowing spin, the Frisbee's forward motion, and the higher air pressure along the flat broad side of the platter as it's settling down.

LIFTOFF

The Frisbee can soar along a straight horizontal line for long distances because of lift. We can demonstrate this once again by putting a hand out the window of a moving car. Holding your hand upright and flat against the oncoming airflow, the air resistance and drag was obvious.

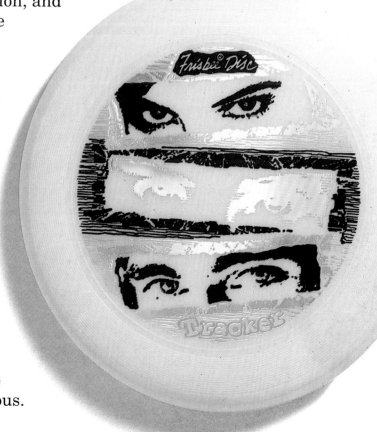

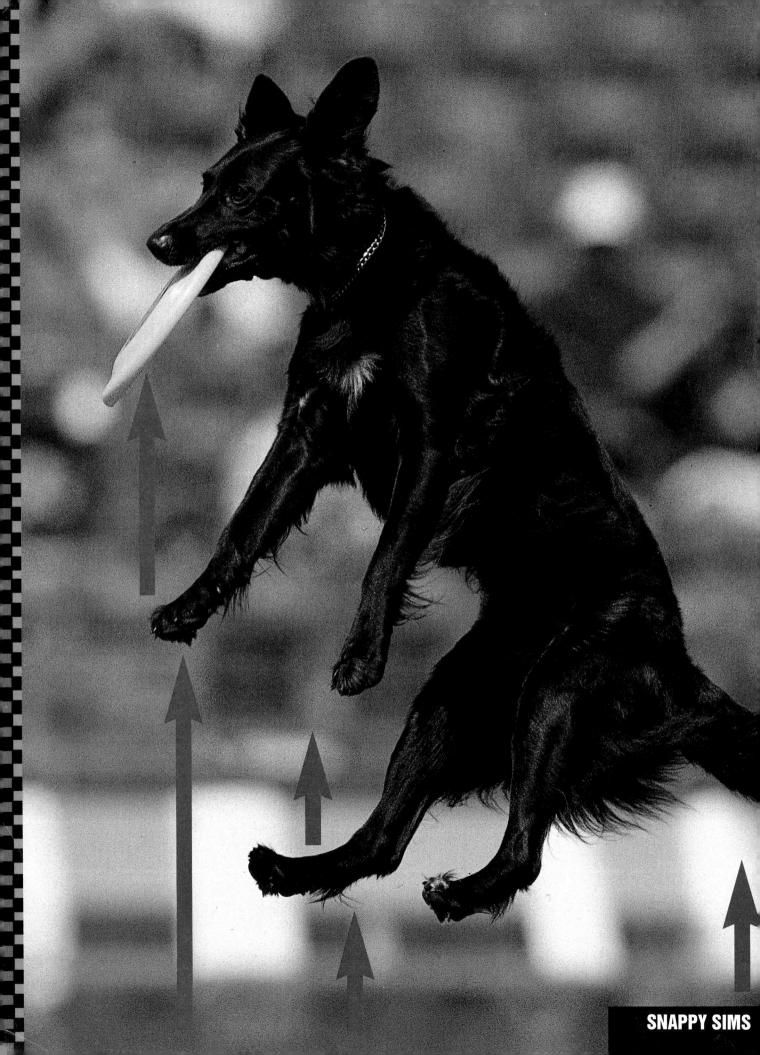

SNAPPY SIMS

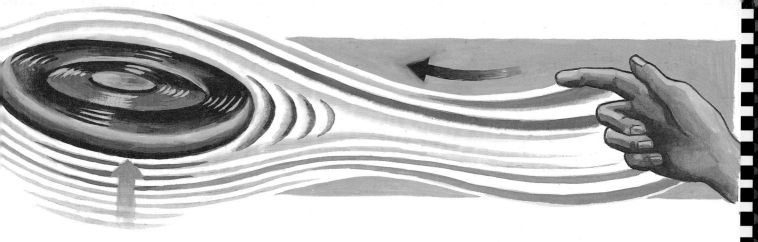

This time, if you angle your hand so that it is almost flat, with just a slight upward angle, you can feel the lift drive your hand upward. The angle of your hand makes the air flow faster over the top of it and slower beneath it. This is what happens to the Frisbee. Greater air pressure coming from underneath gives the platter its lift.

As long as a Frisbee is thrown so it flies with its flat side facing the ground and a slight angle up, it doesn't matter which side of the Frisbee is pointed up. These simple aerodynamic principles are also used in designing airplane wings.

SPINNING SAUCER

Spin is what allows a Frisbee to remain flat throughout its flight. Without spin, a Frisbee would tumble through the air, dipping and diving like a kite without a tail. These twists and tosses encountered by a nonspinning Frisbee or a kite are called torques. These same torques are what can cause a football to wobble as it's moving down field. If you stick your hand back outside the car window, you can feel the torques trying to twist your hand. Much like a discus, the Frisbee counteracts these twists and tumbles with spin.

When the Frisbee spins, air pressure remains even both over it and under it. This allows the Frisbee to stay flat on straight flights. Spin also allows the Frisbee to maintain a constant banked angle on curved flights to maintain a steady lift throughout its flight. Because the majority of a Frisbee's weight is in its outer edges, the faster it spins, the better it holds its path. That is, of course, until the elements of drag slow it enough so that gravity takes over and begins pulling it back to earth.

What we have been talking about are normal flights of the Frisbee. But if you have ever played with a Frisbee, you know normal flights are only half the fun. In spite of the fact that spin helps the Frisbee maintain its stable flight, if the angle that the Frisbee is pointed changes, the air pressure on the two broad sides of the Frisbee switch, and its flight becomes very unpredictable. And, it might even twist and crash.

Hyzer Angle— sideways angle of release for level flight.

Lines of Headrick— circular ridges on Frisbee edge.

Bernoulli's Plate— named for Daniel Bernoulli and his equation describing lift.

The Slope of Schultz— the curve of the Frisbee.

The Bump of Boggio— the center bump on a Frisbee.

Kukuk's Ridge— the bottom ridge of a Frisbee, named for Harry J. Kukuk, executive director of the International Frisbee Association.

DOGS IN PLAY

Enough serious talk. Let's talk about something completely silly—the aerodynamics of Frisbee-catching dogs. Absolutely no scientific studies have been done to calculate the aerodynamics of dog bodies in flight. So let's make something up. It is probably safe to assume that these canine Frisbee chompers defy air resistance by the lift of their ears. Of course, unlike a baseball, there is no spin associated with a leaping dog, so one can only guess that a dog's flight time is limited by the drag against its nonaerodynamic body and the pull of gravity.

In looking at these critters in flight, one might think that it is the dog's tail that acts as a stabilizing force against air resistance. But from all nonscientific evidence available, that would seem to say that the tail was wagging the dog. Until further studies are done, we should probably just accept the marvel of dogs in flight—and the Frisbees they catch so gracefully.

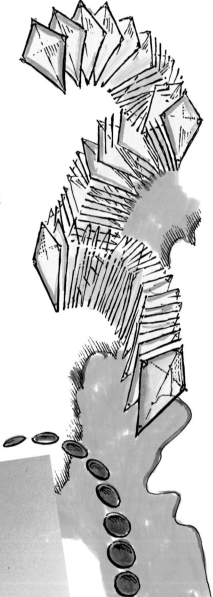

THE AUTHOR

40

AFTERWORD

Most sports are affected by forces that are invisible. They might keep a baseball from flying out of the ballpark, or cause a football to be intercepted and returned for a touchdown. These invisible forces affect the way balls sail, float, and ultimately bounce. And they affect how far or how high athletes' bodies can remain aloft.

It is safe to say that the games we play would be very different if it weren't for the aerodynamic forces that govern them. In fact, if they didn't exist, who knows, Carl Lewis may still be airborne on his gravity-defying attempt to break the new long jump record.

GLOSSARIZED INDEX

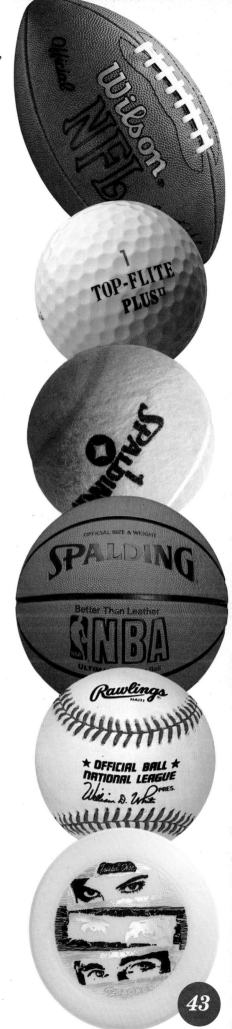

BOOKS FOR YOUNG READERS AGES 8 AND UP

from John Muir Publications

X-ray Vision Series

Each title in the series is 8½" × 11", 48 pages, $9.95, paperback, with four-color photographs and illustrations and written by Ron Schultz.

Looking Inside the Brain

Looking Inside Cartoon Animation

Looking Inside Sports Aerodynamics

Looking Inside Sunken Treasure

Looking Inside Telescopes and the Night Sky

Masters of Motion Series

Each title in the series is 10¼" × 9", 48 pages, $9.95, paperback, with four-color photographs and illustrations.

How to Drive an Indy Race Car
David Rubel

How to Fly a 747
Tim Paulson

How to Fly the Space Shuttle
Russell Shorto
(avail. 12/92)

The Extremely Weird Series

All of the titles in the Extremely Weird Series are written by Sarah Lovett, are 8½" × 11", 48 pages, and $9.95 paperbacks.

Extremely Weird Bats

Extremely Weird Birds

Extremely Weird Endangered Species

Extremely Weird Fishes

Extremely Weird Frogs

Extremely Weird Insects

Extremely Weird Primates

Extremely Weird Reptiles

Extremely Weird Sea Creatures

Extremely Weird Spiders

Other Titles of Interest

Habitats
Where the Wild Things Live
Randi Hacker and Jackie Kaufman
8½" × 11", 48 pages, color illustrations
$9.95 paper

The Indian Way
Learning to Communicate with Mother Earth
Gary McLain
Paintings by Gary McLain
Illustrations by Michael Taylor
7" × 9", 114 pages, two-color illustrations
$9.95 paper

Kids Explore America's Hispanic Heritage
Westridge Young Writers Workshop
7" × 9", 112 pages, illustrations
$7.95 paper

Rads, Ergs, and Cheeseburgers
The Kids' Guide to Energy and the Environment
Bill Yanda
Illustrated by Michael Taylor
7" × 9", 108 pages, two-color illustrations
$12.95 paper

The Kids' Environment Book
What's Awry and Why
Anne Pedersen
Illustrated by Sally Blakemore
7" × 9", 192 pages, two-color illustrations
$13.95 paper
For Ages 10 and Up

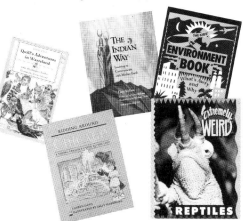

The Quill Hedgehog Adventures Series

Green fiction for young readers. Each title in the series is written by John Waddington-Feather and illustrated by Doreen Edmond.

Quill's Adventures in the Great Beyond
Book One
5½" × 8½", 96 pages, $5.95 paper

Quill's Adventures in Wasteland
Book Two
5½" × 8½", 132 pages, $5.95 paper

Quill's Adventures in Grozzieland
Book Three
5½" × 8½", 132 pages, $5.95 paper

The Kidding Around Travel Series

All of the titles listed below are 64 pages and $9.95 except for *Kidding Around the National Parks of the Southwest* and *Kidding Around Spain*, which are 108 pages and $12.95.

Kidding Around Atlanta

Kidding Around Boston

Kidding Around Chicago

Kidding Around the Hawaiian Islands

Kidding Around London

Kidding Around Los Angeles

Kidding Around the National Parks of the Southwest

Kidding Around New York City

Kidding Around Paris

Kidding Around Philadelphia

Kidding Around San Diego

Kidding Around San Francisco

Kidding Around Santa Fe

Kidding Around Seattle

Kidding Around Spain

Kidding Around Washington, D.C.